Table Of Contents

Chapter 1: Understanding the Crisis

The Statistics Behind Male Suicide

The statistics surrounding male suicide are stark and unsettling, shedding light on a critical public health issue that demands urgent attention. Globally, men are three to four times more likely to die by suicide than women, a trend consistent across various cultures and demographics. In the United States, the Centers for Disease Control and Prevention (CDC) reported that men accounted for approximately 79% of all suicide deaths in 2019. This disproportionate rate raises important questions about the underlying factors contributing to male suicide and highlights the need for targeted prevention strategies.

Various risk factors contribute to the elevated suicide rates among men. Mental health disorders, particularly depression and anxiety, play a significant role, often exacerbated by societal expectations that discourage men from expressing vulnerability or seeking help. Economic factors, such as unemployment and financial strain, also correlate strongly with suicidal behavior in men. Additionally, men are more likely to use lethal means in suicide attempts, resulting in a higher completion rate.

Understanding these factors is crucial for developing effective interventions that address the specific needs of men.

Demographic data reveals important nuances within the statistics. While younger men (ages 15-24) face significant risks, middle-aged men, particularly those between 45 and 54, have the highest rates of suicide. This age group often grapples with life transitions, such as career changes, relationship breakdowns, and the pressures of fatherhood, which can contribute to feelings of hopelessness. Furthermore, male veterans exhibit a particularly high suicide rate, underscoring the need for specialized support for men who have served in the armed forces and may be dealing with trauma and reintegration challenges.

Cultural and societal influences also play a critical role in male suicide rates. Traditional masculinity norms often promote stoicism and discourage emotional expression, creating barriers for men seeking help. This stigma can lead to a reluctance to discuss mental health issues, further isolating individuals in distress. Addressing these cultural attitudes is essential for encouraging men to seek support and fostering an environment where mental health can be openly discussed without fear of judgment.

Effective prevention strategies must be multifaceted, targeting not only the individual but also the community and societal structures that contribute to the crisis. Initiatives such as mental health education programs, support groups for men, and campaigns that challenge harmful stereotypes can create a more supportive environment. Additionally, training for healthcare providers to recognize signs of distress in men and provide appropriate resources is vital. By combining statistical insights with practical solutions, society can begin to address the unseen crisis of male suicide and work towards a future where all men have access to the help they need.

Sociocultural Factors Contributing to Male Mental Health

Sociocultural factors play a crucial role in shaping male mental health, influencing how men perceive themselves, express emotions, and seek help. Traditional masculinity norms often dictate that men should be stoic, self-reliant, and emotionally reserved. These societal expectations can lead to a reluctance to acknowledge mental health struggles, as vulnerability is often seen as a weakness. Consequently, many men may suffer silently, feeling that they must uphold a façade of strength. This cultural pressure not only limits emotional expression but also discourages open discussions about mental health, perpetuating stigma and isolation.

The impact of societal expectations extends into various aspects of life, including fatherhood and parenting. Men often grapple with the pressure to be the primary breadwinner while also being present and engaged fathers. This dual expectation can create a significant emotional burden, leading to stress and anxiety. As men navigate their roles, they may feel inadequate if they cannot fulfill these societal standards, which can further exacerbate mental health issues. Support systems that encourage open dialogue about the challenges of fatherhood and provide resources for emotional well-being are essential for mitigating these pressures.

Moreover, male victims of domestic violence face unique sociocultural challenges that can significantly affect their mental health. Society often overlooks the experiences of men in abusive situations, leading to feelings of shame and helplessness. This lack of recognition can prevent men from seeking help and support, leaving them trapped in a cycle of silence. Advocacy for male victims must address these sociocultural barriers, emphasizing that seeking help is a sign of strength rather than weakness. Creating awareness about male victimization can encourage more men to come forward and access the resources they need for recovery.

Men's rights in family law also intersect with mental health, as the outcomes of custody battles and divorce can have profound psychological effects on fathers. The perception that men are less capable of nurturing or are often sidelined in custody decisions can contribute to feelings of inadequacy and despair. As men navigate these challenges, it is vital to advocate for equitable treatment within family law systems, ensuring that their rights are upheld and that they receive support during these transitions. This advocacy can help alleviate the mental health toll associated with family disputes.

Finally, addressing male suicide rates requires a multifaceted approach that encompasses sociocultural factors. Suicide prevention strategies must consider the stigmas surrounding male vulnerability and the cultural narratives that discourage emotional expression. Programs aimed at promoting mental health awareness among men should focus on creating safe spaces where they can share their experiences without judgment. By fostering an environment that encourages dialogue and support, society can begin to dismantle the harmful stereotypes that contribute to male mental health crises, ultimately paving the way for healthier outcomes and reduced suicide rates.

The Silence Surrounding Male Suffering

The silence surrounding male suffering is a pervasive issue that often goes unnoticed in societal discourse. Traditional notions of masculinity have ingrained the belief that men must remain stoic and composed, leading many to suppress their emotions and vulnerabilities. This cultural expectation creates an environment where men feel they cannot openly express their pain or seek help, ultimately contributing to the alarming rates of male suicide. Understanding this silence is crucial for addressing the mental health crisis faced by men and developing effective prevention strategies.

Men are often socialized to view emotional expression as a sign of weakness. From a young age, boys are taught to "toughen up," which discourages them from discussing their feelings or seeking support when they encounter challenges. This internalized belief not only stifles their emotional growth but also isolates them during critical times of distress. The fear of judgment or ridicule can lead to a cycle of suffering in silence, where men grapple with their struggles alone, further exacerbating feelings of hopelessness and despair.

The implications of this silence extend to various aspects of men's lives, including fatherhood and parenting. Many fathers feel pressure to be the strong, unyielding figure in their children's lives, often neglecting their own emotional needs. This self-neglect can hinder their ability to be present and engaged parents, ultimately affecting their children's well-being. Advocacy for men's mental health is essential, as it empowers fathers to acknowledge their struggles and seek support, fostering healthier family dynamics and breaking the cycle of emotional suppression.

Moreover, the silence surrounding male suffering is particularly pronounced in discussions of domestic violence. Male victims often face stigma that discourages them from coming forward, fearing they will not be believed or will be viewed as less masculine. This silence not only perpetuates their suffering but also obscures the reality of male victimization, making it difficult to develop adequate support systems and resources for those in need. Addressing this issue requires a shift in societal perceptions and increased awareness of the complexities of male experiences.

To combat the silence surrounding male suffering, it is imperative to create inclusive spaces for men to share their experiences and seek help. Encouraging open dialogues about mental health, challenging traditional gender norms, and providing resources tailored to men can significantly contribute to reducing stigma. By fostering an environment where men feel safe to express their emotions, societies can take meaningful steps towards preventing male suicide and promoting overall mental well-being. Addressing this silence is not only vital for individual men but is also a crucial component in building healthier communities.

Chapter 2: The Importance of Mental Health Awareness

Redefining Masculinity and Mental Health

Redefining masculinity in the context of mental health involves challenging traditional norms and stereotypes that often dictate how men are expected to behave. Historically, masculinity has been associated with strength, stoicism, and emotional restraint. This narrow definition can lead to detrimental outcomes for men who struggle with mental health issues, as they may feel the need to suppress their emotions or avoid seeking help. By broadening the definition of masculinity to include vulnerability, emotional expression, and the pursuit of mental well-being, society can create an environment where men feel safe to address their mental health needs without fear of judgment or stigma.

The impact of redefining masculinity on mental health becomes particularly evident when examining the barriers men face in seeking help. Many men internalize the belief that asking for help is a sign of weakness, which can prevent them from accessing essential mental health services. This reluctance is compounded by societal pressures that equate masculinity with self-sufficiency and independence. By promoting a new narrative that values help-seeking behavior as a strength rather than a weakness, advocates can encourage men to prioritize their mental health and seek out the resources they need to thrive.

Fatherhood and parenting advocacy also play a critical role in redefining masculinity in relation to mental health. As societal expectations shift, fathers increasingly find themselves navigating the complexities of parenting while managing their own mental health. Engaging fathers in conversations about emotional well-being and encouraging them to model healthy behaviors for their children can foster a more supportive environment for future generations. By promoting active involvement in parenting and emotional expression, society can help create a cycle of openness that benefits both men and their families.

Men's rights in family law is another critical aspect of this discussion, as it intersects with mental health in significant ways. Navigating family law issues can be emotionally taxing, particularly for men who may feel marginalized or misunderstood within the legal system. Addressing these concerns requires a holistic approach that acknowledges the unique challenges men face, including mental health struggles that can arise during divorce or custody disputes. By advocating for policies that support men's mental health within the family law framework, we can help reduce the stress and anxiety that often accompany these situations, ultimately lowering the risk of suicidal ideation among men.

Lastly, understanding the prevalence of male victims of domestic violence is essential in redefining masculinity and its relationship to mental health. Male victims often face additional barriers when seeking help, including stigma and a lack of appropriate resources. By acknowledging that men can be victims and promoting services that cater to their specific needs, we can create a more inclusive approach to mental health advocacy. This shift not only helps men find the support they need but also challenges harmful stereotypes about masculinity, paving the way for a more nuanced understanding of male experiences and mental health. Through these combined efforts, we can work towards reducing male suicide rates and fostering a culture that champions mental health for all.

Breaking Down Stigmas

Breaking down stigmas surrounding male mental health is crucial in addressing the alarming rates of suicide among men. Traditionally, societal norms have often dictated that men should be stoic, strong, and self-reliant, discouraging them from expressing vulnerability or seeking help. These ingrained beliefs have created an environment where men feel they must suffer in silence, fearing judgment or ridicule for admitting to their struggles. By challenging these outdated stereotypes, we can foster a culture that encourages open conversations about mental health and normalizes the act of seeking support.

Education plays a vital role in dismantling these stigmas. Initiatives aimed at raising awareness about men's mental health issues can help to inform both men and women about the unique challenges men face. Workshops, community programs, and media campaigns can provide valuable information about recognizing mental health symptoms and the importance of seeking help. When individuals understand that mental health issues can affect anyone, regardless of gender, they are more likely to support their friends, family members, and peers in seeking the help they need.

Moreover, creating safe spaces for men to express their feelings is essential in breaking down these stigmas. Support groups, therapy sessions, and mentorship programs tailored for men can provide environments where they feel comfortable discussing their experiences without fear of judgment. These spaces can help men realize that they are not alone in their struggles and that vulnerability is a sign of strength, not weakness. Encouraging participation in these initiatives can significantly alter perceptions and create a supportive network for men dealing with mental health challenges.

Changing the narrative around masculinity is another critical component of breaking down stigmas. Promoting a more inclusive definition of masculinity that embraces emotional expression and vulnerability can empower men to seek help. By highlighting positive role models who exemplify these traits, we can inspire men to redefine what it means to be strong. This shift in perspective can help dismantle the harmful beliefs that prevent many men from reaching out for assistance and can lead to healthier coping strategies and improved mental well-being.

Finally, advocating for policy changes that support men's mental health is essential in addressing the systemic issues contributing to these stigmas. This includes increasing funding for mental health services, implementing educational programs in schools and workplaces, and ensuring that mental health resources are accessible to all men. By addressing the structural barriers that hinder men from seeking help, we can create a more supportive environment that not only breaks down stigmas but also promotes overall mental health awareness and prevention strategies. Through these collective efforts, we can work towards reducing the suicide rates among men and fostering a society where mental health is openly discussed and prioritized.

The Role of Media in Shaping Perceptions

The media plays a crucial role in shaping societal perceptions, particularly concerning sensitive issues such as male mental health and suicide. Through the various platforms it utilizes, including news outlets, social media, and entertainment, media influences public discourse and can either reinforce or challenge existing stereotypes about masculinity and mental health. This influence is particularly significant in the context of male suicide, where societal narratives often depict men as stoic and emotionally resilient. Such portrayals can discourage men from seeking help or discussing their struggles, ultimately contributing to the stigma surrounding male vulnerability.

News coverage of male suicide often focuses on sensationalism rather than providing a nuanced understanding of the underlying causes. When stories prioritize shock value over empathy, they may inadvertently perpetuate harmful stereotypes and create a climate of fear rather than support. For instance, depicting male suicide solely as a result of individual failures neglects the systemic issues, such as economic instability, social isolation, and lack of adequate mental health resources that disproportionately affect men. A more responsible media approach would involve highlighting these broader societal factors, thereby fostering a more compassionate public understanding of the challenges faced by men.

Social media has emerged as a double-edged sword in this context. On one hand, it provides a platform for advocacy, allowing men to share their experiences and connect with others facing similar challenges. Campaigns aimed at raising awareness about male mental health can reach extensive audiences, breaking down barriers to discussion and encouraging those in need to seek support. On the other hand, social media can also amplify negative stereotypes and promote harmful behaviors, particularly through the spread of memes or narratives that trivialize mental health issues. Striking a balance between positive discourse and the risks of misinformation is essential for fostering a supportive environment for men.

Furthermore, the representation of men in entertainment media significantly impacts public perceptions. Films and television shows often depict male characters in rigid roles that emphasize toughness and emotional suppression. These portrayals can shape audience expectations about masculinity, leading to a reluctance to acknowledge vulnerability as a natural human experience. By promoting diverse and authentic representations of male characters grappling with mental health issues, entertainment media can challenge traditional notions of masculinity and encourage viewers to adopt a more empathetic perspective.

In conclusion, the media's role in shaping perceptions surrounding male suicide and mental health is both powerful and complex. It has the potential to either entrench harmful stereotypes or foster understanding and empathy. As advocates for men's mental health, it is crucial to engage with media narratives critically and promote responsible coverage that emphasizes the importance of emotional expression and support. By doing so, society can begin to dismantle the barriers preventing men from seeking help and create a more informed and compassionate approach to addressing male suicide and its prevention.

Chapter 3: Fatherhood and Its Impact on Mental Health

The Challenges of Modern Fatherhood

The challenges of modern fatherhood are multifaceted, shaped by evolving societal expectations and the pressures of contemporary life. Fathers today are often caught between traditional roles and the push for more involved parenting. This shift has led to a re-examination of what it means to be a father, with many men striving to balance work, family responsibilities, and their own mental health. The expectation to be both a provider and an active participant in child-rearing can create stress and anxiety, particularly when societal norms still lean towards traditional masculinity, which often discourages emotional expression and vulnerability.

One major challenge is the lack of support systems for fathers. While maternal support networks have gained traction, paternal resources remain limited. Many fathers report feelings of isolation and inadequacy, particularly in the early stages of parenting. The stigma surrounding men's mental health prevents many from seeking help, leading to a dangerous cycle where feelings of depression or anxiety go unaddressed. Fathers may feel they must shoulder their burdens alone, which can exacerbate feelings of distress and contribute to a decline in mental health.

Fathers often grapple with the realities of family law, which can disproportionately affect men's rights in custody arrangements. Many men face systemic biases that can leave them feeling marginalized and powerless in the legal system. This sense of injustice can lead to heightened stress and frustration, impacting not only their mental health but their ability to engage meaningfully in their children's lives. The emotional toll of navigating these challenges can be profound, pushing some fathers towards despair and, in the most tragic cases, suicidal ideation.

The issue of male victims of domestic violence is another critical aspect that complicates modern fatherhood. Many men are reluctant to speak out about their experiences due to societal perceptions that undermine their victimhood. This silence can lead to feelings of shame, further isolating them from potential support systems. When fathers are victims of domestic violence, their ability to parent effectively and maintain a healthy relationship with their children is severely compromised, which can perpetuate cycles of trauma and instability within families.

Ultimately, addressing the challenges of modern fatherhood requires a comprehensive approach that includes increased awareness of men's mental health issues, advocacy for equitable family law practices, and the development of supportive communities for fathers. By fostering environments where men can express their feelings and seek help without stigma, society can mitigate the risks of isolation and despair that contribute to rising male suicide rates. It is essential to recognize the critical role of fathers in families and to provide them with the resources they need to thrive, not only for their well-being but for the benefit of their children and future generations.

Parenting and Emotional Wellbeing

Parenting plays a crucial role in shaping emotional wellbeing, especially for fathers who may face unique challenges in their relationships with their children and partners. Understanding the dynamics of fatherhood is essential for fostering a supportive environment where emotional expression is encouraged. Fathers often grapple with societal expectations that dictate how they should behave, sometimes leading them to suppress their emotions. Addressing these pressures can significantly impact not only their wellbeing but also the emotional health of their children, creating a cycle that influences future generations.

Emotional wellbeing in parenting is intrinsically linked to communication within the family unit. Fathers who feel comfortable expressing their thoughts and feelings set a precedent for their children, promoting open dialogue about emotions. This environment is vital in combating the stigma surrounding male vulnerability. Encouraging children to articulate their feelings helps them develop emotional intelligence and resilience, equipping them to handle life's challenges more effectively. Supportive parenting can diminish the risk of mental health issues, including anxiety and depression, that are prevalent among both boys and girls.

The legal and social frameworks surrounding family law often impact fathers' emotional wellbeing. Many men experience feelings of isolation and helplessness during custody battles or when navigating complex family dynamics. Advocacy for fathers' rights is essential to ensure that they are not marginalized in these processes. By promoting equitable family law practices, society can help alleviate some of the pressures that contribute to emotional distress. When fathers feel empowered to participate actively in their children's lives, it enhances their sense of purpose and connection, contributing to better mental health outcomes.

Additionally, addressing the issue of male victims of domestic violence is vital for a comprehensive approach to parenting and emotional wellbeing. Men often face stigmatization when seeking help or reporting abuse, leading to unaddressed trauma that can affect their parenting capabilities. Creating awareness and providing resources for male victims can help them reclaim their emotional health, which, in turn, influences their interactions with their children. By fostering an environment where all victims of domestic violence can seek support without fear of judgment, we can promote healthier family dynamics and enhance overall wellbeing.

In conclusion, the intersection of parenting and emotional wellbeing is a critical area that warrants attention in the conversation surrounding male mental health. By advocating for supportive family structures, equitable legal frameworks, and open emotional expression, we can create an environment that nurtures both fathers and their children. This holistic approach not only aids in reducing male suicide rates but also cultivates a generation that values emotional health and resilience. Addressing these issues is not merely about preventing crisis, but about fostering a thriving, emotionally aware community where all members can flourish.

Supporting Fathers in Crisis

Supporting fathers in crisis is a crucial aspect of addressing the broader issue of male mental health and suicide prevention. Many fathers face unique challenges that can significantly impact their mental well-being, particularly during periods of crisis. These challenges can include financial stress, relationship breakdowns, and the struggle to balance work and family responsibilities. By creating an environment that acknowledges these pressures and provides targeted support, we can help fathers navigate their difficulties and reduce the risk of suicidal thoughts and behaviors.

One of the key elements in supporting fathers in crisis is recognizing the stigma surrounding male vulnerability. Society often promotes the notion that men should be stoic and self-reliant, which can discourage fathers from seeking help when they need it most. Campaigns aimed at normalizing discussions about mental health and encouraging men to share their struggles can play a vital role in breaking down these barriers. Awareness initiatives can help fathers understand that it is not only acceptable but necessary to seek support, whether through friends, family, or professional services.

Access to mental health resources tailored specifically for fathers is essential. Many existing programs focus broadly on mental health without addressing the unique experiences of fathers. Developing support groups that cater to fathers, providing them with a safe space to express their feelings and share their experiences, can foster community and understanding. Moreover, integrating mental health education into parenting classes can equip fathers with the tools they need to recognize signs of mental distress in themselves and others, promoting early intervention.

Family law can also significantly impact fathers in crisis, particularly in cases of separation or divorce. Advocating for fair treatment in family court systems is critical in ensuring that fathers retain meaningful relationships with their children. This advocacy not only benefits the fathers but also contributes to the emotional well-being of their children. Legal support services that understand the challenges faced by fathers can provide guidance and representation, alleviating some of the stress associated with navigating family law issues.

Lastly, addressing male victims of domestic violence is an often-overlooked aspect of supporting fathers in crisis. Men can be victims of domestic abuse, yet their experiences are frequently minimized or ignored. Providing resources and support specifically for male victims is essential in helping them escape abusive situations and rebuild their lives. By ensuring that fathers in crisis have access to comprehensive support systems that address their mental health, legal rights, and safety, we can create a more inclusive approach to male suicide prevention and overall well-being.

Chapter 4: Men's Rights in Family Law

Understanding Legal Challenges for Men

Understanding the legal challenges that men face is crucial in addressing the broader issue of male suicide and mental health. Various legal systems often reflect societal biases that can impact men profoundly, especially in family law, domestic violence cases, and health care access. These challenges can contribute to feelings of helplessness and isolation, which are known risk factors for suicide. By exploring these legal hurdles, we can better understand how they intersect with men's mental health and advocate for necessary reforms.

In family law, men frequently encounter biases that can affect custody arrangements and child support obligations. The prevailing assumption in many jurisdictions is that women are more suitable custodians for children, often leading to unfavorable outcomes for fathers seeking to maintain relationships with their children. The emotional toll of these experiences can exacerbate feelings of inadequacy and depression among men, making it essential to advocate for fairer legal standards that recognize the importance of both parents in a child's life.

Men are also disproportionately affected by domestic violence yet often lack adequate legal protections. Societal stigma can prevent male victims from seeking help, fearing they will not be taken seriously by authorities or that they will be ridiculed. Legal responses to domestic violence tend to focus predominantly on female victims, further alienating men who may be suffering in silence. Addressing this imbalance is vital in creating a support system that encourages male victims to come forward and seek the assistance they need.

Health care access presents another significant legal challenge for men. Many health care systems are not adequately designed to address men's specific health issues or psychological needs. Men often face barriers when trying to access mental health services, including stigma and a lack of resources tailored to them. The legal frameworks governing health care can inadvertently perpetuate these barriers, making it essential to advocate for policies that promote equitable access to mental health care and preventative services for men.

Ultimately, understanding and addressing these legal challenges is a crucial step in tackling the unseen crisis of male suicide. By highlighting the intersection of law and mental health, we can foster greater awareness among policymakers and the public about the unique struggles men face. Advocacy for legal reforms that ensure fairness in family law, protection for male victims of domestic violence, and improved health care access can contribute significantly to reducing male suicide rates and promoting overall well-being for men.

The Impact of Divorce and Custody Battles

Divorce and custody battles represent profound challenges that can significantly impact men's mental health and overall well-being. The emotional turmoil associated with the dissolution of a marriage often leads to feelings of loss, rejection, and helplessness. For many men, the struggle to maintain meaningful relationships with their children during and after divorce can exacerbate these feelings, leading to increased stress and anxiety. The societal perception of men as primary breadwinners and providers intensifies the pressure, as they may feel they are failing in their roles, which can contribute to a decline in mental health.

The legal processes surrounding divorce and custody can be daunting and are often skewed against men. Many fathers face systemic biases that can affect custody arrangements, often resulting in reduced parenting time and strained father-child relationships. This situation can lead to feelings of inadequacy and frustration, as men grapple with the loss of day-to-day involvement in their children's lives. The emotional toll of navigating a family court system that may not favor their interests can lead to feelings of alienation and despair, further compounding mental health issues.

Financial implications of divorce also play a critical role in the psychological well-being of men. The often exorbitant costs associated with legal representation, child support, and alimony can create financial strain that adds to the stress of an already difficult situation. Many men report feelings of helplessness when faced with the prospect of losing their financial stability alongside their familial connections. This financial pressure can lead to negative coping mechanisms, such as substance abuse, which further deteriorates mental health and increases the risk of suicidal thoughts and behaviors.

Additionally, the stigma surrounding men's mental health and the reluctance to seek help can leave many fathers isolated during these challenging times. Societal expectations often dictate that men remain stoic and self-reliant, which can prevent them from accessing support services that could mitigate the impact of divorce and custody battles. This isolation can be detrimental, as it deprives men of the opportunity to express their feelings and seek help, potentially leading to a downward spiral in mental health and an increased risk of suicide.

Addressing the impact of divorce and custody battles on men requires a multifaceted approach that recognizes the unique challenges they face. Advocacy for equitable family law practices is essential to ensure that men's rights are protected and that they can maintain meaningful relationships with their children. Increased awareness of men's mental health issues, along with accessible support networks, can encourage men to seek help rather than suffer in silence. By fostering an environment where men feel supported and understood, we can mitigate the unseen crisis of male suicide and ultimately contribute to healthier outcomes for fathers and families alike.

Advocating for Fair Treatment in Family Courts

Family courts play a crucial role in determining the outcomes of familial relationships and parental responsibilities, yet they often reflect systemic biases that can leave men feeling marginalized. Advocating for fair treatment in these courts is essential for promoting mental health and well-being among men, particularly fathers who may face uphill battles in custody and support disputes. The perception that family courts are inherently biased against men can create a sense of hopelessness, which, coupled with the pressures of fatherhood and societal expectations, can lead to increased mental health struggles and even suicidal ideation.

One of the key issues in family courts is the presumption of maternal custody, which can undermine fathers' rights and their involvement in their children's lives. This presumption can lead to a lack of equitable treatment for fathers, resulting in feelings of alienation and inadequacy. When men are denied meaningful involvement in their children's upbringing, it can exacerbate existing mental health issues and contribute to a sense of loss and despair. Advocating for fair treatment involves challenging these outdated presumptions and promoting a more balanced view of parenting roles, which recognizes the value that fathers bring to their children's lives.

Legal representation is another critical factor in advocating for fair treatment in family courts. Many men find themselves navigating complex legal waters without adequate support, which can lead to unfavorable outcomes. Access to legal resources that understand men's rights and the nuances of family law is essential. Organizations that specialize in providing legal aid to men facing family court issues can play a pivotal role in leveling the playing field. By equipping men with the resources they need, advocates can help ensure that their voices are heard and respected in courtrooms, which is vital for their mental health and overall well-being.

Furthermore, raising awareness about male victims of domestic violence is an essential component of advocating for fair treatment in family courts. Men often face stigma and disbelief when they come forward as victims, which can deter them from seeking help. By addressing these issues head-on, advocates can help create a more supportive environment where all victims are recognized and treated with dignity. This includes pushing for policies that acknowledge and protect male victims, ensuring they receive the support they need in family court proceedings, which can significantly impact their mental health and future safety.

Finally, advocacy efforts must extend beyond the courtroom to encompass broader societal changes. By challenging stereotypes and misconceptions about masculinity, advocates can foster a cultural shift that encourages men to engage in discussions about their rights and mental health. Community initiatives that promote fatherhood, support systems for male victims, and mental health resources tailored for men are crucial. When men feel supported and empowered to advocate for themselves, it can lead to improved mental health outcomes and a decrease in suicide rates among this demographic. Emphasizing fair treatment in family courts is a vital step in addressing the unseen crisis of male suicide and promoting a healthier, more equitable society for all.

Chapter 5: Recognizing Male Victims of Domestic Violence

The Reality of Male Victimhood

The concept of male victimhood often exists in the shadows of societal norms and expectations. Men are frequently portrayed as strong, resilient figures who are not supposed to show vulnerability or seek help. This cultural narrative can lead to the underreporting of male victimization in various forms, including domestic violence, sexual abuse, and mental health struggles. Recognizing that men can indeed be victims is crucial for fostering a more inclusive understanding of these issues. By addressing male victimhood openly, society can create a more supportive environment that encourages men to seek help without fear of judgment.

One of the most significant areas where male victimhood is overlooked is domestic violence. While the prevalent narrative often focuses on women as victims, many men endure physical and emotional abuse from their partners. Studies indicate that a considerable number of men experience domestic violence, yet they are less likely to report it, fearing stigma or disbelief. This underreporting not only perpetuates the myth that men cannot be victims but also leaves those who are suffering without the necessary support and resources. Addressing this disparity is essential for both raising awareness and providing appropriate interventions for male victims.

Mental health is another critical area impacted by the reality of male victimhood. The societal pressure on men to conform to traditional masculine ideals can inhibit their willingness to discuss emotional pain or seek psychological help. This reluctance is compounded when men face victimization, as they may feel additional shame or embarrassment. Consequently, many men suffering from depression, anxiety, or trauma go untreated, leading to dire consequences, including increased risk of suicide. It is vital for mental health advocates to emphasize that seeking help is a sign of strength, not weakness, and that male victims deserve the same level of support and understanding as their female counterparts.

Fatherhood and parenting advocacy also intersect with the issue of male victimhood. Fathers who experience domestic violence or other forms of victimization face unique challenges when navigating family law systems. Often, these men may find themselves marginalized or disbelieved, which can further complicate their roles as parents. The impact of victimization on parenting can be profound, affecting a father's mental health and ability to engage with their children. Advocating for the rights of fathers in family law, while also addressing their experiences as victims, is crucial for ensuring that all parents can provide a safe and nurturing environment for their children.

Ultimately, addressing male victimhood is not just about recognizing the struggles men face but also about fostering a more comprehensive approach to mental health and well-being. By inclusively addressing male experiences, society can dismantle harmful stereotypes and encourage open dialogues about vulnerability. This shift is necessary not only for improving support systems for male victims but also for reducing the overall rates of male suicide. Acknowledging and validating the reality of male victimhood is a vital step in creating a more equitable and understanding society, where all individuals, regardless of gender, can seek help and find healing.

Barriers to Seeking Help

Barriers to seeking help for mental health issues are particularly pronounced among men, contributing significantly to the rising rates of male suicide. Traditional societal norms often dictate that men should be stoic, self-reliant, and emotionally resilient, leading many to view vulnerability as a weakness. This cultural conditioning discourages open discussions about mental health and creates an environment where seeking help is perceived as a failure. As a result, many men suffer in silence, grappling with feelings of depression, anxiety, and isolation without the support they desperately need.

Fear of stigma is another significant barrier that prevents men from seeking assistance. Men may worry about how peers, family, and coworkers will perceive them if they disclose their struggles. This fear can be particularly acute in environments that prioritize toughness and emotional concealment. The stigma surrounding mental health issues can lead to internalized shame, where men believe they must navigate their challenges alone. This perception not only exacerbates their struggles but also reinforces harmful stereotypes about masculinity, further isolating them from potential support systems.

Access to resources can also pose a challenge for men seeking help. In many communities, mental health services are underfunded and not easily accessible, particularly for those in rural or marginalized areas. Men may find it difficult to locate services that cater specifically to their needs or may encounter long waiting times for appointments. Additionally, some may lack knowledge about available resources or how to navigate the healthcare system effectively. This inaccessibility can lead to frustration and hopelessness, further discouraging men from reaching out for help.

Another barrier arises from the misconception that seeking help is only necessary in extreme situations. Many men believe they must hit rock bottom before they can justify seeking support, which can result in a crisis that might have been preventable. This mentality can be particularly detrimental in the context of fatherhood, where men may prioritize their responsibilities to their families over their own mental health. By normalizing the idea that proactive mental health care is essential, rather than a last resort, we can encourage men to seek help earlier and more frequently.

Lastly, a lack of targeted outreach and support programs specifically for men can hinder their willingness to seek assistance. Many mental health services are designed with a one-size-fits-all approach, which may not resonate with male clients. Developing programs that understand and address the unique experiences and challenges faced by men can help break down these barriers. By fostering environments that encourage open dialogue and offer tailored resources, we can empower men to prioritize their mental health, ultimately reducing the stigma and incidence of male suicide.

Support Systems for Male Survivors

Support systems for male survivors of trauma, particularly those who have experienced domestic violence or mental health struggles, are vital in promoting healing and recovery. Unlike traditional narratives that often overlook men's experiences, recognizing the unique challenges faced by male survivors is essential for effective support. These systems must be multifaceted, incorporating professional mental health services, peer support networks, and community resources that resonate with men's specific needs. By fostering environments where men can openly share their experiences without stigma, we create pathways for healing and resilience.

Professional mental health services play a crucial role in the support system for male survivors. Access to trained therapists who understand the complexities of male trauma is essential. Many men may feel uncomfortable seeking help due to societal expectations of masculinity, which can discourage vulnerability. Therefore, therapy models that focus on empowerment, resilience, and practical coping strategies can be particularly effective. Additionally, integrating approaches like cognitive-behavioral therapy and mindfulness can help male survivors develop essential skills to manage their emotions and navigate their trauma.

Peer support networks are equally important for male survivors, as they provide a safe space for men to connect with others who share similar experiences. Support groups specifically tailored for men can help break down feelings of isolation and shame. These groups can facilitate open discussions about challenges unique to male survivors, such as societal pressures or feelings of inadequacy. Through shared experiences, participants can validate each other's feelings and foster a sense of camaraderie that promotes healing. Encouraging men to share their stories can also empower them to take control of their narratives, transforming their experiences from sources of pain into catalysts for personal strength.

Community resources that address the broader context of male survivors' lives are also critical. Organizations that focus on men's health issues, family law rights, and advocacy for male victims of domestic violence can provide essential information and support. By creating partnerships between mental health professionals and community organizations, a comprehensive support network can be established. This collaboration can ensure that male survivors have access to legal resources, counseling, and preventive care, addressing their needs from multiple angles and promoting overall well-being.

Finally, raising awareness about male survivors and their support systems is crucial for societal change. Advocacy efforts should aim to dismantle stigmas surrounding male vulnerability and encourage open discussions about men's mental health. By promoting educational initiatives that focus on the realities of male trauma and the importance of support systems, we can begin to shift cultural perceptions. As society becomes more informed about the unique challenges faced by male survivors, it will be better equipped to provide the necessary support, ultimately contributing to lower suicide rates and healthier outcomes for men across all demographics.

Chapter 6: Addressing Men's Health Issues

Common Health Concerns Affecting Men

Common health concerns affecting men encompass a range of physical and mental health issues that can significantly impact their quality of life and overall well-being. Heart disease stands as a leading health threat for men, often attributed to lifestyle factors such as poor diet, lack of exercise, and high stress levels. Regular check-ups, awareness of family health history, and lifestyle modifications can play a crucial role in prevention. Men should be encouraged to engage in routine health screenings and adopt heart-healthy habits, including a balanced diet and regular physical activity, to mitigate risks associated with cardiovascular diseases.

Mental health issues are another significant concern for men, who often face societal pressures to conform to traditional masculine norms that discourage emotional expression. Conditions such as depression and anxiety frequently go unreported and untreated, leading to devastating consequences. The stigma surrounding mental health can prevent men from seeking help, making it imperative to foster an environment where discussing mental health is normalized. Support systems, including therapy and peer support groups, can provide men with the necessary tools to address their mental health challenges, ultimately reducing the risk of suicide.

Sexual health problems, including erectile dysfunction and low testosterone levels, are also prevalent among men, particularly as they age. These issues can lead to emotional distress, affecting self-esteem and relationships. It is essential for men to understand that these health concerns are common and treatable. Open discussions with healthcare providers can lead to effective treatment options, allowing men to regain confidence in their sexual health and overall vitality. Preventative care, including regular screenings for sexually transmitted infections and prostate health, remains critical.

Men are also at a heightened risk for substance abuse, which often serves as a coping mechanism for underlying mental health issues. Alcohol and drug abuse can exacerbate other health problems, creating a vicious cycle that further deteriorates physical and mental health. Public health initiatives aimed at educating men about the dangers of substance abuse and promoting healthier coping strategies are vital. Encouraging participation in activities that foster connection and community can help mitigate feelings of isolation, which often contribute to substance dependency.

Lastly, awareness of domestic violence against men is crucial in addressing their health concerns. Male victims often face societal disbelief and stigma that can prevent them from seeking help. It is essential to create supportive environments where men feel safe to disclose their experiences and access necessary resources. Advocacy for men's rights in family law, as well as increased visibility of male victims in support programs, can contribute to breaking the cycle of silence and creating a more inclusive approach to health and wellness. By addressing these common health concerns, society can take significant strides toward reducing male suicide rates and fostering a healthier, more supportive environment for men.

Preventative Care and Health Education

Preventative care and health education play a pivotal role in addressing the factors contributing to male suicide rates. This segment of health strategy emphasizes the importance of early intervention and proactive health management, particularly in the context of men's mental health. Men often face societal pressures that discourage them from seeking help or discussing their emotional well-being. By promoting preventative care, we can encourage men to engage with healthcare systems, recognize early signs of mental distress, and seek support before situations escalate.

Health education tailored to men's unique challenges is equally essential. This education can take many forms, including community workshops, online resources, and peer support groups. Topics such as the importance of regular health check-ups, understanding mental health issues, and recognizing the signs of depression and anxiety can equip men with the knowledge they need to take charge of their well-being. Furthermore, integrating discussions about fatherhood and parenting can help men understand how their mental health impacts their families, thereby fostering a sense of responsibility that encourages them to prioritize their health.

Advocating for men's rights in family law is another critical aspect of preventative care and health education. Men often experience unique challenges during family disputes, which can exacerbate mental health issues. By educating men about their rights and the resources available to them—such as legal counseling and support networks—individuals can feel empowered to navigate these complex situations. This empowerment can reduce feelings of isolation and helplessness, which are significant risk factors for suicidal thoughts and behaviors.

Moreover, addressing male victims of domestic violence must be a priority in preventative health strategies. Many men suffer in silence due to stigma and a lack of resources directed towards them. Educational initiatives that raise awareness about male victimization can help dismantle stereotypes and create a more inclusive support system. By providing resources and safe havens for men who have experienced domestic violence, we can address underlying psychological trauma and prevent the mental health deterioration that often leads to suicidal ideation.

Ultimately, a comprehensive approach to preventative care and health education must include collaboration among healthcare providers, community organizations, and policymakers. By fostering environments where men feel safe to discuss their health, seek help, and access educational resources, we can significantly reduce the stigma surrounding men's mental health. This collective effort not only addresses immediate health concerns but also contributes to long-term cultural shifts that prioritize mental well-being, ultimately leading to a decrease in male suicide rates.

The Role of Healthcare Providers in Male Health

Healthcare providers play an essential role in addressing male health, particularly in the context of mental health and suicide prevention. Men often face societal pressures that discourage them from seeking help, which can lead to a reluctance to discuss their emotional and psychological well-being. Healthcare providers must create an environment where men feel safe and supported to express their concerns. This involves not only being aware of the unique challenges men face but also actively engaging them in conversations about their mental health. The stigma associated with mental health issues in men can be diminished through empathetic communication and by normalizing discussions around emotional struggles.

One of the primary responsibilities of healthcare providers is to educate men about the importance of regular check-ups and preventive care. Many men prioritize work and family responsibilities over their health, often neglecting necessary medical evaluations and screenings. By promoting awareness of common male health issues, such as heart disease, prostate cancer, and mental health conditions, providers can encourage men to take proactive steps towards their well-being. Educational initiatives can include workshops, informational pamphlets, and community outreach that focus specifically on men's health concerns, emphasizing the importance of early detection and intervention.

In addition to physical health, healthcare providers must advocate for mental health resources tailored to men. This includes recognizing the signs of depression, anxiety, and stress, which may manifest differently in men compared to women. Training healthcare providers to understand these differences can lead to more accurate diagnoses and effective treatment plans. Furthermore, integrating mental health screenings into routine health assessments can help identify men who may be at risk for suicide or other serious mental health issues, allowing for timely interventions and support.

Healthcare providers also have a critical role in addressing the impact of societal factors on male health. Many men experience challenges related to fatherhood, employment, and relationships that can contribute to feelings of inadequacy and isolation. By providing support and resources that address these social determinants of health, providers can help men navigate these complexities. This may involve referrals to counseling services, support groups, or educational programs aimed at enhancing parenting skills and promoting healthy relationships. A holistic approach to male health considers not only the physical aspects but also the emotional and social elements that contribute to overall well-being.

Finally, healthcare providers can be advocates for policy changes that benefit men's health on a broader scale. This includes pushing for legislation that addresses male suicide rates, enhances mental health resources, and promotes awareness of men's health issues within the community. By collaborating with organizations focused on men's rights, mental health advocacy, and family law, healthcare providers can help shape a supportive framework that prioritizes male health. Creating a culture that values men's well-being is crucial for reducing stigma, improving access to care, and ultimately fostering a society where men feel empowered to seek help and support when needed.

Chapter 7: Strategies for Suicide Prevention

Identifying Warning Signs

Identifying warning signs of male suicide is crucial for effective prevention and intervention. Men often exhibit a range of behaviors and emotional cues that may indicate they are struggling. These signs can be subtle, making it essential for friends, family, and colleagues to be vigilant and informed. Common warning signs include withdrawal from social activities, changes in mood, and an increase in risky behaviors. When a man who typically engages in social interactions suddenly isolates himself, or when he displays extreme irritability or anger, these can be red flags that warrant attention.

Another significant indicator is changes in sleep patterns and appetite. A man who starts to experience insomnia or excessive sleeping may be confronting underlying mental health issues. Similarly, drastic changes in eating habits, whether an increase or decrease, can signal distress. These physical manifestations often accompany emotional struggles, yet they can go unnoticed if those around him are not attuned to the potential implications. It is vital to foster an environment where discussions about mental health are normalized, allowing individuals to express their challenges openly.

Additionally, men may express feelings of hopelessness or worthlessness, which are critical signs of emotional turmoil. When statements reflecting a lack of purpose or a belief that life is no longer worth living arise, they should be taken seriously. It is essential to understand that these feelings can be part of a larger pattern of depressive symptoms. Encouraging conversations about mental health can help to create a supportive atmosphere, where men feel comfortable sharing their thoughts and emotions without judgment.

Substance abuse is another prevalent warning sign that often accompanies suicidal thoughts. Many men may turn to alcohol or drugs as a means to cope with emotional pain, leading to a downward spiral in their mental health. Increased substance use can impair judgment and exacerbate feelings of despair. Recognizing this pattern is vital for family and friends, as it can serve as an entry point for intervention. Support from loved ones can help redirect men toward healthier coping mechanisms and therapeutic resources.

Finally, direct talk about suicide should never be ignored. If a man openly discusses suicidal thoughts or intentions, it is imperative to take such statements seriously. Engaging in a compassionate dialogue about these feelings can provide an opportunity for connection and support. It is essential to approach these conversations with empathy, ensuring that the individual feels heard and understood. By identifying these warning signs and responding appropriately, we can play a crucial role in preventing male suicide, fostering a culture of awareness, and promoting mental health support for men in need.

Creating Supportive Environments

Creating supportive environments is crucial in addressing the rising rates of male suicide and fostering mental health awareness. These environments can be established within the family, workplace, and community settings, providing men with the necessary support systems to discuss their struggles and seek help when needed. By creating a culture that values open communication and emotional expression, we can mitigate the stigma often associated with men's mental health issues and encourage proactive measures for prevention.

In family settings, parents and guardians play a pivotal role in shaping a child's understanding of emotional health. Fathers, in particular, can influence their sons by modeling emotional openness and resilience. Encouraging boys to express their feelings and seek help when they face difficulties can set a strong foundation for future mental health. Family activities that promote bonding and dialogue, such as family meetings or shared hobbies, can help create an atmosphere where emotional well-being is prioritized and normalized.

Workplaces also present a significant opportunity for fostering supportive environments. Employers can implement mental health initiatives that focus on awareness and education, ensuring that male employees feel safe discussing their mental health challenges. Providing resources such as counseling services, support groups, and mental health days can demonstrate a commitment to employee well-being. Training for management on recognizing signs of distress in male employees can also cultivate a culture of support and understanding, leading to improved mental health outcomes.

Community involvement is essential in creating supportive environments beyond the confines of home and work. Local organizations can host workshops and events focused on male mental health awareness, providing forums for discussion and resource sharing. Programs that specifically target male victims of domestic violence can help break down barriers and provide necessary support. The engagement of community leaders and influencers in advocating for men's mental health can also inspire more men to seek help and participate in supportive networks.

Finally, addressing systemic issues within family law and societal perceptions of masculinity is critical in shaping supportive environments. Advocating for men's rights in family law can help ensure fair treatment and resources for fathers, reducing feelings of isolation and despair. By recognizing the unique challenges faced by men in various life situations, society can work towards dismantling harmful stereotypes. Ultimately, creating supportive environments is a multifaceted approach that requires commitment from families, workplaces, communities, and institutions to effectively combat the unseen crisis of male suicide.

Community and Online Resources for Help

Community and online resources play a vital role in addressing male suicide and promoting mental health awareness. Men often face unique challenges that hinder their willingness to seek help, including societal expectations and stigma. Building a supportive community is essential for creating safe spaces where men can express their feelings and experiences without fear of judgment. Local support groups, community centers, and mental health workshops can offer men the chance to connect with others who understand their struggles. These gatherings not only provide emotional support but also encourage men to share coping strategies and resources that have been beneficial in their journeys.

Online resources have become increasingly important in the digital age, offering anonymity and accessibility to those in need. Websites dedicated to men's mental health provide valuable information about common issues, coping mechanisms, and professional help. Forums and social media groups allow men to communicate openly about their experiences and to find camaraderie among peers. These platforms can be particularly beneficial for those who may feel isolated or reluctant to seek help in person. They foster a sense of belonging and remind individuals that they are not alone in their struggles, which can be a critical step in addressing mental health issues.

In addition to general mental health resources, there are specific organizations and hotlines tailored to men's issues. Organizations focused on men's rights in family law and male victims of domestic violence provide essential support and advocacy. These resources not only offer guidance on navigating legal challenges but also promote awareness of the unique difficulties men face in these situations. By raising awareness and providing targeted support, these organizations contribute to a broader understanding of men's mental health and the factors that can lead to suicidal thoughts and behaviors.

Fatherhood and parenting advocacy are also crucial components of community support for men. Many fathers experience stress related to parenting, work-life balance, and societal expectations regarding masculinity. Resources that focus on fatherhood can help men navigate these challenges by providing parenting tips, emotional support, and networking opportunities with other fathers. By fostering strong relationships within the community, men can experience a sense of purpose and belonging that can significantly improve their mental well-being.

Lastly, preventive care and health resources are vital in addressing men's health issues. Health education campaigns that target men emphasize the importance of regular check-ups, physical activity, and mental health screenings. Encouraging men to prioritize their health can lead to early intervention and reduce the risk of severe mental health crises. By utilizing community and online resources, men can access the information and support necessary to make informed decisions about their health, ultimately contributing to a decrease in suicide rates and a healthier, more resilient male population.

Chapter 8: Building a Supportive Network

The Importance of Peer Support

Peer support plays a crucial role in addressing the mental health challenges faced by men, particularly in the context of suicide prevention. Men often face societal pressures to conform to traditional notions of masculinity, which can discourage them from seeking help or expressing vulnerability. As a result, many may suffer in silence, feeling isolated and unsupported. Establishing peer support networks can provide a vital lifeline, offering men a platform to share their experiences, challenges, and coping strategies in a safe and understanding environment. This collective approach not only fosters camaraderie but also helps to normalize conversations around mental health, making it easier for men to seek help when needed.

One of the key benefits of peer support is its ability to break down the barriers of stigma associated with mental health issues. Men are frequently taught to be stoic and self-reliant, leading to a reluctance to discuss emotional struggles. Through peer support groups, men can witness firsthand that they are not alone in their experiences. Hearing stories from peers who have faced similar challenges can create a sense of belonging and understanding, reducing feelings of alienation. This shared experience can encourage men to open up about their own difficulties and seek professional help, ultimately leading to improved mental health outcomes.

Moreover, peer support can empower men by providing them with tools and techniques to handle stress, anxiety, and depression. Peer-led initiatives often include workshops, discussions, and activities that focus on coping mechanisms and resilience-building strategies. These programs can teach men how to communicate their feelings effectively, recognize warning signs in themselves and others, and develop a proactive approach to mental health. By equipping men with these skills, peer support not only addresses immediate concerns but also contributes to long-term emotional well-being.

In addition to improving individual mental health, peer support can also foster a sense of community among men. In an era where social connections can be fleeting, establishing meaningful relationships through shared experiences can be incredibly beneficial. This sense of community provides men with opportunities to connect, collaborate, and support one another in their journeys. It can also lead to increased awareness of issues such as male victims of domestic violence and the challenges faced in family law, allowing for collective advocacy and a stronger voice in policy discussions that affect men's rights and well-being.

Ultimately, the importance of peer support in addressing male suicide and mental health cannot be overstated. By creating inclusive environments where men feel safe to express their emotions and seek support, we can dismantle the stigma associated with mental health struggles. Encouraging peer interactions not only aids in individual healing but also strengthens the fabric of our communities, paving the way for a more compassionate understanding of men's mental health issues. As we continue to address the unseen crisis of male suicide, prioritizing peer support will be a critical strategy in fostering resilience and encouraging help-seeking behavior among men.

Engaging Men in Mental Health Initiatives

Engaging men in mental health initiatives is crucial for addressing the alarming rates of male suicide and promoting overall mental well-being. Traditionally, mental health discussions have often excluded men or framed them in ways that feel inaccessible or stigmatizing. To foster an environment where men feel comfortable seeking help, it is essential to understand the unique barriers they face. Societal norms often dictate that men should be stoic and self-reliant, which can lead to reluctance in discussing emotions or seeking support. Mental health initiatives must therefore be tailored to resonate with men, encouraging them to embrace vulnerability as a strength rather than a weakness.

One effective approach to engage men in mental health initiatives is through community-based programs that emphasize peer support. Men are more likely to open up about their struggles when they feel they are in a safe, judgment-free space with others who share similar experiences. Creating support groups or workshops specifically for men can help dismantle the stigma surrounding mental health while promoting a sense of camaraderie. These environments allow for honest discussions about issues such as stress, depression, and anxiety, providing men with tools and language to articulate their feelings and experiences.

Incorporating male role models into mental health initiatives can also significantly enhance engagement. Fathers, community leaders, and public figures who openly discuss their mental health journeys can serve as powerful advocates for change. By sharing their own experiences with mental health challenges, these role models can inspire other men to seek help and normalize conversations around mental health. Campaigns that highlight testimonials from men who have experienced mental health struggles can create a ripple effect, encouraging others to step forward and share their stories.

Educational outreach is another critical component in engaging men with mental health initiatives. Programs that focus on preventative care and early intervention can help men recognize the signs of mental health issues in themselves and others. Workshops tailored to specific groups, such as fathers or men in high-stress professions, can provide relevant strategies for managing mental health. When men are equipped with knowledge about mental health resources and coping strategies, they are more likely to take proactive steps toward seeking help and supporting their peers.

Finally, advocacy for men's rights in family law and attention to male victims of domestic violence are essential pieces of the puzzle in engaging men in mental health initiatives. Many men may feel marginalized within these contexts, leading to feelings of isolation and hopelessness. By addressing these issues and promoting a more inclusive understanding of mental health that considers the specific challenges men face, initiatives can create a supportive framework that resonates with a broader male audience. Ultimately, prioritizing men's mental health and involving them in the conversation will be vital in reducing the stigma and rates of male suicide, leading to healthier communities.

Successful Programs and Models

Successful programs and models addressing male suicide and its prevention have emerged as critical tools in combating this pressing issue. These initiatives often draw on comprehensive strategies that incorporate mental health services, community engagement, and targeted outreach efforts. One noteworthy model is the "Man Up" campaign, which focuses on breaking down the stigma surrounding men's mental health. By promoting open discussions and providing resources tailored specifically for men, this program creates safe spaces for individuals to express their struggles and seek help without fear of judgment.

Another effective approach is the incorporation of peer support networks. Programs like "BroTalk" empower men by connecting them with trained peers who have experienced similar challenges. These networks foster a sense of community and belonging, which is essential for individuals who may feel isolated due to their mental health issues. By normalizing conversations about emotional well-being and providing accessible support, these programs significantly reduce the barriers men face when seeking help.

Additionally, integrating mental health education into schools and workplaces has proven to be an effective strategy. Programs that train educators and employers to recognize the signs of mental distress in men can lead to early intervention and support. Workshops and seminars that focus on emotional intelligence and coping mechanisms equip individuals with the tools necessary to navigate their mental health. This proactive approach not only aids in prevention but also promotes a culture that values mental well-being as a fundamental aspect of overall health.

Family-focused interventions also play a crucial role in preventing male suicide. Initiatives that emphasize fatherhood and parenting advocacy provide resources for men to strengthen their familial relationships and improve their emotional resilience. Programs that offer parenting classes and support groups encourage fathers to engage actively in their children's lives, fostering a nurturing environment that benefits both parents and children. This connection can alleviate feelings of isolation and inadequacy that often contribute to mental health struggles.

Finally, it is essential to highlight the role of policy advocacy in creating systemic change. Successful programs often include efforts to reform family law and increase awareness of male victims of domestic violence. By addressing these issues within the legal framework, advocates can ensure that men's rights are recognized and respected. Comprehensive strategies that combine grassroots efforts with legislative advocacy are vital for creating a supportive environment that prioritizes men's mental health and reduces suicide rates. Through the implementation of these successful models, communities can work towards a future where every man feels valued, supported, and empowered to seek help when needed.

Chapter 9: Advocating for Change

Policy Changes to Support Male Mental Health

Policy changes aimed at supporting male mental health are crucial in addressing the alarming rates of male suicide and promoting overall well-being. A multifaceted approach is needed to create an environment where men feel comfortable seeking help and accessing mental health resources. This includes reforming existing policies and implementing new initiatives that specifically target the unique challenges men face. By doing so, society can foster a culture that prioritizes mental health for all genders while ensuring that men's specific needs are not overlooked.

First and foremost, mental health services must be made more accessible to men. This can be accomplished by increasing funding for community-based mental health programs that cater specifically to men. Such programs can focus on male-oriented therapeutic approaches, offering group therapy sessions and workshops that emphasize shared experiences and camaraderie. Additionally, integrating mental health education into schools and workplaces can raise awareness about the importance of mental health and encourage men to seek help without stigma. By normalizing conversations around mental health, policies can help dismantle the barriers that prevent men from accessing critical support.

Moreover, policies that promote work-life balance and parental leave are essential in addressing men's mental health issues, particularly for fathers. Research indicates that fatherhood can significantly impact men's mental health, and policies that support equal parental leave for both mothers and fathers can alleviate stress and promote healthy family dynamics. Encouraging workplaces to adopt flexible working arrangements can also help fathers manage their responsibilities, reducing the feeling of being overwhelmed. When fathers are supported in their roles, they are more likely to engage positively with their children and maintain their mental well-being.

Addressing male victims of domestic violence is another crucial element of policy change. Historically, support systems for domestic violence have primarily focused on female victims, often leaving male victims without adequate resources. By implementing policies that recognize and address male victimization, society can create a more inclusive support network. This includes establishing shelters that cater to male victims, training law enforcement to respond sensitively to male victimization, and providing mental health resources specifically tailored to their experiences. Such changes can empower men to seek help and ultimately reduce the stigma surrounding male victimization.

Finally, promoting research and data collection specifically focused on male mental health is vital for informing policy changes. Governments and organizations should invest in studies that explore the unique mental health challenges faced by men, as well as effective intervention strategies. By understanding the specific factors contributing to male mental health issues, policymakers can develop targeted programs that address these concerns. This evidence-based approach will not only enhance the effectiveness of mental health initiatives but also ensure that resources are allocated where they are needed most, ultimately contributing to a significant reduction in male suicide rates.

Community Involvement and Activism

Community involvement and activism play a crucial role in addressing the complex issues surrounding male suicide and mental health. When men feel connected to their communities, they are more likely to seek help and support during challenging times. Engaging in community initiatives can foster a sense of belonging and purpose, which are essential elements for mental well-being. By creating spaces where men can openly discuss their feelings and experiences, communities can reduce the stigma surrounding mental health issues and encourage more individuals to share their struggles without fear of judgment.

One effective way to promote male mental health awareness is through organized events that focus on education and support. Workshops, seminars, and outreach programs can provide vital information about mental health resources available to men. These events can also feature speakers who share their personal stories of overcoming mental health challenges, demonstrating that recovery is possible. Furthermore, community-led initiatives can empower men to take an active role in their mental health by offering tools and strategies for coping with stress, anxiety, and depression.

Advocacy efforts that target specific issues, such as family law and support for male victims of domestic violence, are essential to creating a more equitable society. By raising awareness about the challenges men face in these areas, communities can push for legislative changes that offer greater protection and resources. This includes advocating for fair treatment in custody disputes, increased funding for support services for male victims, and creating public campaigns that highlight the importance of addressing male-specific issues. Such activism not only benefits individuals but also contributes to a broader cultural shift that acknowledges and addresses the unique challenges men encounter.

Involving men in community service and activism can also serve as a preventive measure against suicide. When men engage in altruistic activities, they often experience increased feelings of self-worth and connection. Volunteering can provide a sense of purpose, reduce feelings of isolation, and create opportunities for building supportive relationships. By emphasizing the importance of giving back to the community, organizations can encourage men to channel their energy into positive actions, which can have a lasting impact on their mental health.

Ultimately, community involvement and activism are vital components in the fight against male suicide. By fostering open conversations, advocating for systemic change, and encouraging proactive engagement, communities can create an environment where men feel supported and empowered to seek help. This comprehensive approach not only addresses the immediate crisis of male suicide but also contributes to a healthier, more resilient society that values the mental well-being of all its members.

The Role of Education in Prevention

Education plays a pivotal role in the prevention of male suicide, serving as a fundamental tool for raising awareness and fostering understanding around mental health issues. It equips individuals with the knowledge necessary to recognize the signs of distress in themselves and others, dispelling the stigmas that often surround discussions of mental health, particularly among men. By integrating mental health education into schools, workplaces, and community programs, society can create an environment where open conversations about emotional struggles are encouraged, rather than suppressed. This proactive approach can help to identify at-risk individuals and provide them with the support they need before crisis situations arise.

In the context of fatherhood and parenting, education can empower fathers to understand their own emotional well-being and the importance of mental health in their role as caregivers. Programs designed to educate men about stress management, coping strategies, and the impact of their mental health on their children can lead to healthier family dynamics. Fathers who are educated about the signs of depression and anxiety are more likely to seek help for themselves, creating a positive feedback loop that benefits both their own health and that of their family. This understanding not only helps to reduce the stigma surrounding mental health but also encourages fathers to model healthy emotional behavior for their children.

Additionally, education on men's rights in family law is essential in preventing feelings of helplessness and despair that can contribute to suicidal thoughts. Many men face significant challenges in navigating family law issues, often feeling marginalized or misunderstood. Providing educational resources that outline their rights and available support systems can empower men to advocate for themselves effectively. When men are informed about their legal rights and the resources available to them, they are more likely to engage positively with the legal system, reducing feelings of isolation and increasing their likelihood of seeking mental health support.

Male victims of domestic violence often experience unique challenges that can lead to increased vulnerability to suicide. Education can play a crucial role in helping men recognize that they are not alone and that there are resources available to assist them. Community education initiatives that focus on the experiences of male victims can help dismantle the stigma that prevents many from seeking help. By raising awareness about the realities of male victimization, communities can foster a more supportive environment, encouraging men to share their experiences and seek the necessary help without fear of judgment.

Finally, education around general men's health issues and preventive care is vital in addressing the broader context of male suicide rates. Many men engage in risky behaviors, neglect their physical health, and avoid seeking medical attention due to societal expectations of masculinity. Comprehensive health education that highlights the importance of regular check-ups, mental health screenings, and healthy lifestyle choices can lead to better overall health outcomes. When men understand the connection between physical health and mental well-being, they are more likely to take proactive steps toward maintaining both, thus reducing the risk of suicide. By fostering a culture of health literacy among men, society can take significant strides toward preventing the unseen crisis of male suicide.

Chapter 10: Moving Forward

Cultivating a Culture of Openness

Cultivating a culture of openness is essential in addressing the pressing issue of male suicide and mental health. This culture encourages men to express their feelings and seek help without the fear of stigma or judgment. In many societies, traditional notions of masculinity often promote emotional suppression and discourage vulnerability. By actively challenging these norms, communities can create safe spaces where men feel empowered to share their struggles and experiences. This shift not only benefits individuals but also fosters stronger relationships and support networks among men, ultimately contributing to a decrease in suicide rates.

One effective strategy in cultivating openness is the implementation of educational programs that focus on emotional literacy. These programs can be integrated into schools, workplaces, and community organizations, teaching men the importance of recognizing and articulating their emotions. Workshops that include role-playing scenarios, discussions about mental health, and strategies for effective communication can equip men with the tools they need to express themselves. By normalizing conversations around mental health, these initiatives can help dismantle the barriers that often prevent men from seeking help when they need it most.

Furthermore, support groups specifically designed for men can play a crucial role in fostering openness. These groups provide a platform for sharing experiences, discussing challenges, and offering peer support. Men who participate in these groups often find solace in knowing they are not alone in their struggles. The shared experience can help reduce feelings of isolation and promote a sense of belonging. Additionally, these groups can be facilitated by trained professionals who understand the unique challenges men face, ensuring a safe environment for honest dialogue.

Creating policies that prioritize mental health resources for men is another vital step in cultivating a culture of openness. Governments and organizations should invest in programs that provide access to mental health services, including counseling and therapy tailored specifically for men. These services should be advertised in ways that resonate with male audiences, utilizing language and imagery that reflect their experiences. By making mental health resources visible and accessible, communities can encourage men to seek help without fear of judgment, ultimately leading to improved mental health outcomes.

Finally, media representation plays a pivotal role in shaping cultural perceptions of masculinity and mental health. By promoting stories that depict men openly discussing their struggles and seeking help, media can challenge harmful stereotypes and inspire others to do the same. Campaigns that highlight male role models who advocate for mental health awareness can change the narrative around masculinity. When men see their peers and public figures embracing vulnerability, it sends a powerful message that seeking help is a strength, not a weakness. Through these combined efforts, cultivating a culture of openness can significantly impact the fight against male suicide and improve overall mental health for men.

Encouraging Men to Seek Help

Encouraging men to seek help is a crucial aspect of addressing the unseen crisis of male suicide. The stigma surrounding mental health often dissuades men from reaching out for support, leading to an alarming number of unaddressed issues. Society traditionally associates masculinity with strength, self-reliance, and emotional restraint, which can create barriers for men when they are confronted with mental health challenges. It is essential to challenge these stereotypes and foster an environment where seeking help is seen as a sign of courage rather than weakness.

Awareness campaigns that specifically target men can play a vital role in changing perceptions around mental health. By utilizing relatable figures, such as athletes, actors, or community leaders, these campaigns can convey messages that resonate with men. Highlighting stories of men who have successfully sought help can serve as powerful testimonials, showing that vulnerability is not synonymous with failure. Furthermore, integrating discussions of mental health into spaces where men naturally congregate, such as sports events or workplaces, can normalize the topic and make it more accessible.

In addition to awareness campaigns, creating support networks tailored to men's needs is essential. These networks can include peer support groups, workshops, and online forums where men can share their experiences in a safe environment. Encouraging open dialogue about mental health in these settings can help dismantle the barriers of isolation and shame. Men must see that they are not alone in their struggles and that it is entirely acceptable to seek assistance from others who understand their experiences.

Fatherhood and parenting advocacy also play a significant role in encouraging men to seek help. Fathers often carry the dual weight of providing for their families while fulfilling emotional roles. By promoting the idea that seeking help improves not only their own well-being but also their capacity to be present and supportive for their children, we can shift the narrative. Parenting programs that incorporate mental health resources can empower fathers to prioritize their mental health, ultimately fostering healthier family dynamics.

Lastly, addressing male victims of domestic violence and their unique challenges is crucial in the conversation about help-seeking behavior. Many men experiencing domestic violence may feel particularly reluctant to reach out due to societal perceptions of masculinity. Providing clear information and accessible resources specifically for male victims can encourage them to seek the help they need. It is vital to ensure that all men understand that they deserve support and that there are safe avenues available for them to receive it. By creating a culture that values emotional health for men, we can begin to see a decline in suicide rates and an increase in overall well-being.

The Vision for a Healthier Future for Men

The vision for a healthier future for men is grounded in a comprehensive understanding of the multifaceted challenges they face. As societal norms evolve, it becomes increasingly crucial to address the hidden struggles that contribute to poor mental health outcomes and a higher risk of suicide among men. This vision encompasses the promotion of open dialogues surrounding men's mental health, recognizing that vulnerability does not equate to weakness. By fostering environments where men feel safe to express their emotions and seek help, we can dismantle the stigma that often surrounds mental health issues.

Advocating for men's rights in various societal contexts, such as family law and domestic violence, is a vital component of this vision. Men often face unique challenges in these areas, and addressing these issues can lead to improved mental health outcomes. Legal frameworks must adapt to ensure fairness and equity, providing men with the support they need during family crises. By creating policies that acknowledge the emotional and psychological toll of these situations, we can help men navigate their circumstances with dignity and respect, ultimately reducing the risk of suicide.

Fatherhood and parenting advocacy play a significant role in shaping the future for men. Encouraging positive father-child relationships not only benefits children but also enhances fathers' mental health and well-being. Support systems for fathers, including parenting classes and mental health resources, can empower them to engage in their children's lives meaningfully. As we emphasize the importance of active fatherhood, we also create opportunities for men to share their experiences, fostering a sense of community and reducing feelings of isolation.

Preventative care and health education tailored specifically for men are critical steps in realizing this vision. Many men neglect their health due to societal pressures or misconceptions about masculinity. By promoting regular health check-ups, mental health screenings, and healthy lifestyle choices, we can significantly reduce the incidence of health issues that contribute to higher suicide rates. Public health campaigns that resonate with men's experiences and challenges can play an essential role in encouraging proactive health management.

Ultimately, the vision for a healthier future for men involves a collective effort from individuals, communities, and institutions. It requires a commitment to creating supportive environments that prioritize mental health awareness and prevention strategies. By advocating for men's rights, promoting positive parenting, and enhancing health care accessibility, we can build a more robust support network for men facing crises. This holistic approach not only addresses immediate needs but also lays the groundwork for a future where men can thrive emotionally, psychologically, and physically, significantly reducing the risk of suicide.

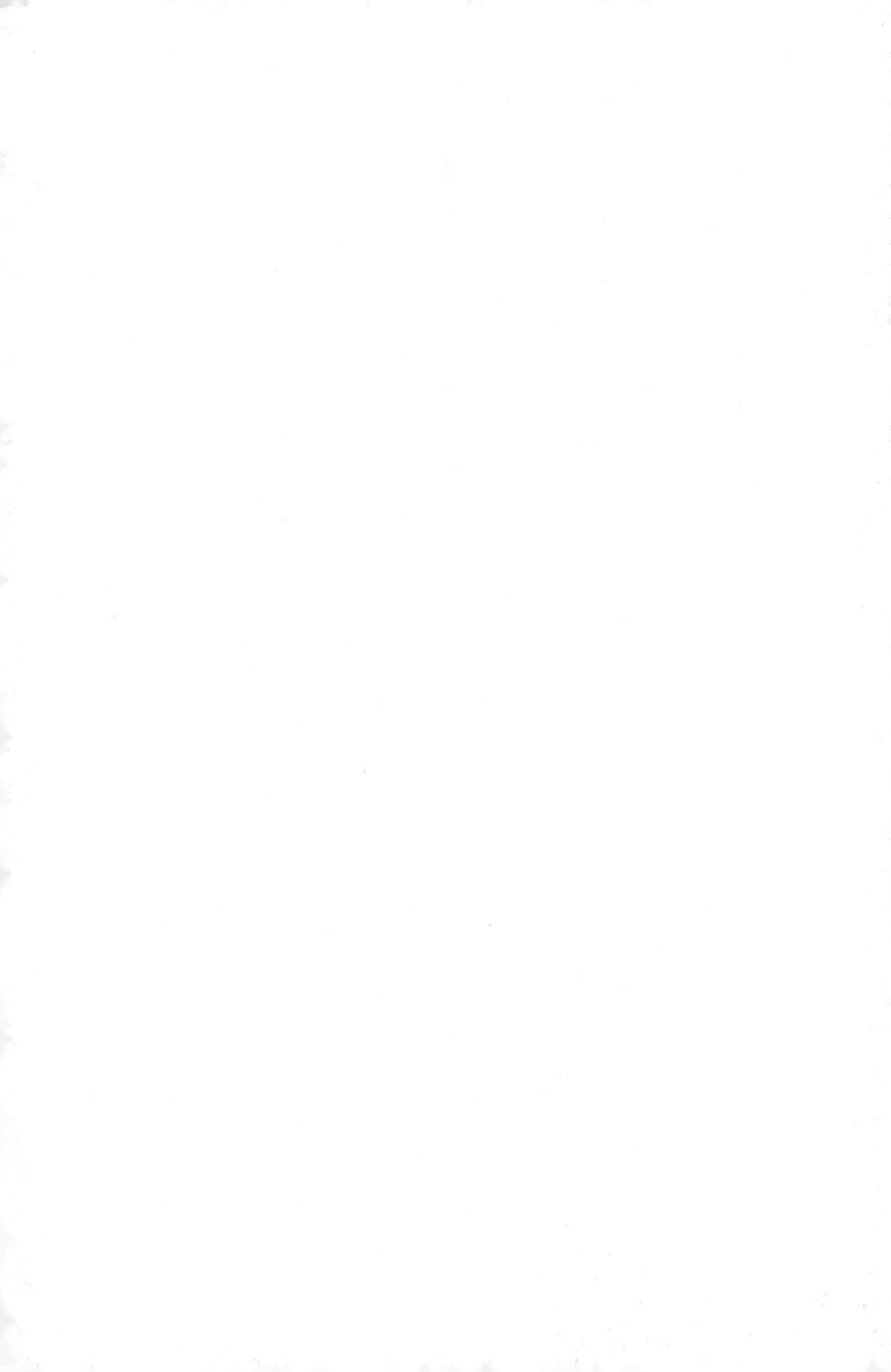